No Gallbladder Diet Cookbook For Beginners

A Comprehensive Guide to Nourishing Recipes, Delicious Living and Optimal Digestive Health and Wellness

Juanita T. Williams

Table of Contents

Turkey Meatballs in Marinara Sauce

Vegetable and Tofu Stir-Fry

Baked Cod with Mediterranean Salsa

Stuffed Bell Peppers with Ground Beef and Rice

Lemon Garlic Shrimp with Zucchini Noodles

Greek Yogurt Chicken Salad

Vegetable Frittata

Stuffed Acorn Squash with Quinoa and Cranberries

Mushroom and Spinach Stuffed Chicken Breast

Black Bean and Corn Salad

Sweet Potato and Turkey Chili

Zucchini Lasagna

Chicken and Vegetable Skewers

Cauliflower Rice Stir-Fry with Shrimp

Vegetarian Lentil Sloppy Joes

Broccoli and Cheddar Quiche

Cabbage and Sausage Skillet

Honey Garlic Glazed Salmon

Eggplant Parmesan

Shrimp and Avocado Salad

Taco-Stuffed Peppers

Mango Salsa Chicken

Lemon Herb Baked Cod

Roasted Brussels Sprouts with Bacon

Turkey and Vegetable Stir-Fry

Mediterranean Quinoa Salad

Turkey and Vegetable Soup

Stuffed Portobello Mushrooms with Quinoa and Spinach

Honey Mustard Baked Chicken

Spinach and Mushroom Quesadillas

Greek Chicken Pita Wraps

Sesame Ginger Tofu Stir-Fry

Caprese Stuffed Chicken

Quinoa-Stuffed Bell Peppers

Tuna and White Bean Salad

Turkey Meatballs with Marinara Sauce

Stuffed Acorn Squash with Quinoa and Cranberries

Zucchini Noodles with Pesto and Cherry Tomatoes

Salmon and Asparagus Foil Packets

Vegetarian Chili

INTRODUCTION

Welcome to the beginning of your journey living without a gallbladder. Whether you've recently undergone surgery or are considering it, understanding how to adapt your diet and lifestyle is crucial for maintaining optimal health and well-being.

Living without a gallbladder may seem daunting at first, but rest assured, millions of people around the world thrive without this small organ. The gallbladder plays a role in storing and releasing bile, a digestive fluid produced by the liver to help break down fats.

Without a gallbladder, bile flows directly from the liver into the small intestine, which can affect digestion, particularly the processing of fats.

However, with the right knowledge and adjustments, you can continue to enjoy a fulfilling and satisfying life post-gallbladder removal. This journey begins with understanding the role of the gallbladder in digestion and how its absence may impact your dietary choices and overall well-being.

Throughout this book, we'll explore practical strategies, delicious recipes, and invaluable tips to support you on your no gallbladder journey. From navigating dietary changes to optimizing nutrient absorption, you'll gain the tools and confidence needed to thrive without a gallbladder.

Let's embark on this journey together, empowering you to embrace your new reality and live life to the fullest without the constraints of gallbladder concerns.

Understanding the No Gallbladder Diet

In order to effectively manage life without a gallbladder, it's essential to have a comprehensive understanding of the no gallbladder diet. This diet focuses on making dietary adjustments to compensate for the absence of the gallbladder and ensure smooth digestion and minimal discomfort.

One of the primary goals of the no gallbladder diet is to minimize the consumption of foods that are high in fat or difficult to digest. Since the gallbladder is responsible for storing and releasing bile to aid in fat digestion, individuals without a gallbladder may experience challenges in digesting fatty foods.

Therefore, it's important to prioritize lean proteins, complex carbohydrates, and healthy fats in your diet.

Additionally, incorporating plenty of fiber-rich foods, such as fruits, vegetables, and whole grains, can help support digestion and promote regular bowel movements.

Fiber aids in the elimination of waste products from the body, which can be particularly beneficial for individuals without a gallbladder who may experience changes in bowel habits.

Moreover, staying hydrated is key to maintaining optimal digestion and overall health. Drinking an adequate amount of water throughout the day helps prevent dehydration and supports the digestion and absorption of nutrients.

Throughout this book, we'll delve deeper into the specifics of the no gallbladder diet, providing you with practical tips, delicious recipes, and expert advice to help you navigate this dietary transition with confidence and ease.

Essential Tips for Success on the No Gallbladder Diet

Transitioning to a no gallbladder diet may initially seem overwhelming, but with the right approach and mindset, you can successfully navigate this dietary change and enjoy optimal health and well-being.

Here are some essential tips to help you succeed on the no gallbladder diet:

1. **Gradually introduce dietary changes**: Instead of making drastic changes overnight, gradually transition to the no gallbladder diet by slowly eliminating high-fat foods and incorporating more

lean proteins, fruits, vegetables, and whole grains into your meals.

2. **Focus on portion control**: While it's important to prioritize nutrient-dense foods, portion control is also key to preventing overeating and minimizing digestive discomfort. Be mindful of portion sizes and listen to your body's hunger and fullness cues.

3. **Prioritize lean proteins**: Opt for lean sources of protein, such as skinless poultry, fish, tofu, and legumes, which are easier to digest than fatty cuts of meat. Incorporating protein-rich foods into your meals helps support muscle health and satiety.

4. **Choose healthy fats**: While it's important to limit your intake of saturated and trans fats, incorporating healthy fats, such as avocados, nuts, seeds, and olive oil, can provide essential nutrients and support overall health.

5. **Stay hydrated**: Adequate hydration is essential for maintaining optimal digestion and overall health, especially for individuals without a gallbladder. Aim to drink plenty of water throughout the day and limit your intake of caffeinated and alcoholic beverages, which can contribute to dehydration.

RECIPES

Grilled Lemon Herb Chicken

Ingredients:
- 4 boneless, skinless chicken breasts
- 2 tablespoons olive oil
- 2 cloves garlic, minced
- One tablespoon of finely chopped fresh herbs, like parsley, thyme, and rosemary
- Juice of 1 lemon
- Salt and pepper to taste

To Prepare :
1. In a bowl, mix together olive oil, minced garlic, chopped herbs, lemon juice, salt, and pepper.
2. Place chicken breasts in a resealable plastic bag and pour the marinade over them. For a minimum of half an hour, seal the bag and place it in the fridge.
3. Preheat the grill to medium-high heat. Once the chicken is fully cooked, remove it from the marinade and grill it for 6 to 8 minutes on each side.

Salmon with Dill Sauce

Ingredients:
- 4 salmon fillets
- 1 tablespoon olive oil
- Salt and pepper to taste
- 1/4 cup plain Greek yogurt
- 1 tablespoon chopped fresh dill
- 1 teaspoon lemon juice

To Prepare :
1. Preheat the oven to 375°F (190°C). Place salmon fillets on a baking sheet lined with parchment paper.
2. Drizzle olive oil over salmon and season with salt and pepper. Bake the salmon for 12 to 15 minutes, or until it is cooked through and flake readily when tested with a fork.
3. In a small bowl, mix together Greek yogurt, chopped dill, and lemon juice. Serve salmon with dill sauce.

Quinoa Stuffed Bell Peppers

Ingredients:
- Cut four bell peppers in half and take out the seeds.
- One cup of cooked quinoa, per package directions
- One can (15 ounces) of rinsed and drained black beans
- One cup of frozen or fresh corn kernels
- 1 cup diced tomatoes
- 1 teaspoon chili powder
- 1/2 teaspoon cumin
- Salt and pepper to taste
- Add-ons: sliced avocado, chopped cilantro, and shredded cheese

To Prepare :
1. Preheat the oven to 375°F (190°C). Put the halves of the bell pepper in a baking dish.
2. In a large bowl, mix together cooked quinoa, black beans, corn, diced tomatoes, chili powder, cumin, salt, and pepper.
3. Spoon quinoa mixture into each bell pepper half. Cover the baking dish with

foil and bake for 25-30 minutes, or until
peppers are tender.

4. Remove foil and sprinkle optional
toppings over stuffed peppers before
serving.

Turkey and Vegetable Stir-Fry

Ingredients:
- 1 pound ground turkey
- 2 tablespoons olive oil
- 2 cloves garlic, minced
- 1 tablespoon grated ginger
- 1 bell pepper, sliced
- 1 cup broccoli florets
- 1 cup sliced mushrooms
- 1/4 cup low-sodium soy sauce
- 1 tablespoon rice vinegar
- 1 teaspoon honey
- Optional: For serving, cooked brown rice or quinoa

To Prepare :

1. Heat olive oil in a large skillet over
medium heat. For one minute, add the
grated ginger and minced garlic and
sauté.

2. Add ground turkey to the skillet and cook until browned, breaking it up with a spatula as it cooks.
3. Add sliced bell pepper, broccoli florets, and sliced mushrooms to the skillet. Cook, stirring regularly, until veggies are tender-crisp.
4. In a small bowl, whisk together soy sauce, rice vinegar, and honey. Pour sauce over turkey and vegetables, stirring to combine.
5. Serve turkey and vegetable stir-fry over cooked brown rice or quinoa, if desired.

Baked Cod with Lemon and Herbs

Ingredients:
- 4 cod fillets
- 2 tablespoons olive oil
- 2 cloves garlic, minced
- 1 tablespoon chopped fresh herbs (such as parsley, dill, and chives)
- Juice of 1 lemon
- Salt and pepper to taste

To Prepare :

1. Preheat the oven to 400°F (200°C). Place cod fillets on a baking sheet lined with parchment paper.
2. In a small bowl, mix together olive oil, minced garlic, chopped herbs, lemon juice, salt, and pepper.
3. Drizzle the herb mixture over the cod fillets, ensuring they are evenly coated.
4. Bake cod in the preheated oven for 12-15 minutes, or until the fish is opaque and flakes easily with a fork.
5. Serve baked cod with additional lemon wedges, if desired.

Vegetable Lentil Soup

Ingredients:

- 1 tablespoon olive oil
- 1 onion, diced
- 2 carrots, diced
- 2 celery stalks, diced
- 2 cloves garlic, minced
- 1 cup dried green or brown lentils, rinsed
- 6 cups vegetable broth
- One can of chopped tomatoes (14 ounces)
- 1 teaspoon dried thyme

- 1 teaspoon dried oregano

- Salt and pepper to taste

- Add-ons: shredded Parmesan cheese and finely chopped fresh parsley

To Prepare :

1. In a large pot set over medium heat, warm the olive oil. Add diced onion, carrots, and celery, and sauté until softened, about 5 minutes.

2. Add minced garlic to the bypot and cook for an additional 1 minute, until fragrant.

3. Stir in rinsed lentils, vegetable broth, diced tomatoes, dried thyme, and dried oregano. Bring soup to a boil, then reduce heat and simmer for 25-30 minutes, or until lentils are tender.

4. Season soup with salt and pepper to taste. Serve hot, garnished with chopped fresh parsley and grated Parmesan cheese, if desired.

Spinach and Feta Stuffed Chicken Breast

Ingredients:
- 4 boneless, skinless chicken breasts
- 2 cups fresh spinach leaves
- 1/2 cup crumbled feta cheese
- 1 clove garlic, minced
- 1 tablespoon olive oil
- Salt and pepper to taste

To Prepare :
1. Preheat the oven to 375°F (190°C). Cut a small pocket into each chicken breast with a sharp knife, taking care not to cut all the way through.
2. In a small skillet, heat olive oil over medium heat. Add minced garlic and sauté for 1 minute, until fragrant. Cook the spinach leaves in the skillet until they begin to wilt.
3. Remove skillet from heat and stir in crumbled feta cheese. Spoon spinach and feta mixture into the pockets of the chicken breasts.

4. Place stuffed chicken breasts on a baking sheet lined with parchment paper. Add pepper and salt to taste.

5. Bake chicken in the preheated oven for 25-30 minutes, or until chicken is cooked through and juices run clear when pierced with a fork.

Mediterranean Chickpea Salad

Ingredients:

- Two cans (15 ounces each) of rinsed and drained chickpeas
- 1 cucumber, diced
- 1 bell pepper, diced
- 1/2 red onion, finely chopped
- 1 cup cherry tomatoes, halved
- 1/4 cup chopped fresh parsley
- 1/4 cup chopped fresh mint
- Juice of 1 lemon
- 2 tablespoons olive oil
- 1 teaspoon dried oregano
- Salt and pepper to taste
- Optional: crumbled feta cheese, olives

To Prepare :

1. In a large bowl, combine chickpeas, diced cucumber, diced bell pepper, chopped red onion, halved cherry tomatoes, chopped parsley, and chopped mint.

2. In a small bowl, whisk together lemon juice, olive oil, dried oregano, salt, and pepper. Drizzle dressing over chickpea mixture, then toss to mix.

3. Serve Mediterranean chickpea salad chilled or at room temperature, garnished with crumbled feta cheese and olives, if desired.

Turkey and Vegetable Skillet

Ingredients:

- 1 pound ground turkey
- 1 tablespoon olive oil
- 1 onion, diced
- 2 cloves garlic, minced
- 1 bell pepper, diced
- 1 zucchini, diced
- 1 cup sliced mushrooms
- 1 teaspoon dried Italian seasoning
- Salt and pepper to taste

- Optional toppings: grated Parmesan cheese, chopped fresh basil

To Prepare :

1. Heat olive oil in a large skillet over medium heat. Add diced onion and minced garlic, and sauté for 2-3 minutes, until softened.
2. Add ground turkey to the skillet and cook until browned, breaking it up with a spatula as it cooks.
3. Stir in diced bell pepper, diced zucchini, sliced mushrooms, dried Italian seasoning, salt, and pepper. Sauté the veggies until they are soft, stirring now and then.
4. Serve turkey and vegetable skillet hot, garnished with grated Parmesan cheese and chopped fresh basil, if desired.

Herb-Roasted Chicken Breast

Ingredients: Chicken breast, olive oil, garlic, rosemary, thyme, salt, pepper.

To Prepare :

Preheat the oven to 375°F (190°C). Rub chicken breast with olive oil, minced garlic, chopped rosemary, thyme, salt, and pepper. Roast in the oven for 25-30 minutes or until cooked through.

Quinoa and Vegetable Stir-Fry

Ingredients:

Quinoa, bell peppers, broccoli, carrots, snap peas, soy sauce, ginger, garlic.

To Prepare :

Cook quinoa according to package instructions. In a pan, stir-fry chopped vegetables with minced ginger and garlic until tender. Add cooked quinoa and soy sauce, toss to combine.

Baked Salmon with Lemon and Dill

Ingredients:

Salmon fillets, lemon, fresh dill, olive oil, salt, pepper.

To Prepare :

Preheat the oven to 400°F (200°C). Place salmon fillets on a baking sheet. Drizzle with olive oil, lemon juice, and sprinkle with chopped dill, salt, and pepper. Bake for 12-15 minutes until salmon is cooked through.

Turkey and Sweet Potato Skillet

Ingredients:

Ground turkey, sweet potatoes, onion, bell peppers, spinach, garlic powder, paprika, salt, pepper.

To Prepare :

In a skillet, brown ground turkey with diced sweet potatoes, onion, and bell peppers. Season with garlic powder, paprika, salt, and pepper. Add spinach and cook until wilted.

Caprese Quinoa Salad

Ingredients:

Quinoa, cherry tomatoes, fresh mozzarella, basil, balsamic glaze, olive oil, salt, pepper.

To Prepare :
Cook quinoa according to package instructions. In a bowl, combine cooked quinoa with halved cherry tomatoes, diced fresh mozzarella, chopped basil, drizzle with balsamic glaze and olive oil. Season with salt and pepper.

Spinach and Feta Stuffed Portobello Mushrooms

Ingredients:
Portobello mushrooms, spinach, feta cheese, garlic, olive oil, salt, pepper.

To Prepare :
Remove stems from portobello mushrooms and brush with olive oil. Cook chopped spinach and minced garlic in a skillet until the spinach wilts. Stuff mushrooms with spinach mixture and crumbled feta cheese. Bake in the oven at 375°F (190°C) for 15-20 minutes.

Lentil and Vegetable Stew

Ingredients:
Lentils, carrots, celery, onion, garlic, diced tomatoes, vegetable broth, bay leaves, thyme, salt, pepper.

To Prepare :
In a large pot, sauté diced onion, carrots, and celery until softened. Add minced garlic and cook for another minute. Stir in lentils, diced tomatoes, vegetable broth, bay leaves, and thyme. Once the lentils are soft, bring to a boil, lower the heat, and simmer for 20 to 25 minutes. Season with salt and pepper.

Turkey Meatballs in Marinara Sauce

Ingredients:
Ground turkey, breadcrumbs, egg, garlic, onion, parsley, marinara sauce, olive oil, salt, pepper.

To Prepare :
In a bowl, combine ground turkey with breadcrumbs, beaten egg, minced garlic, chopped onion, chopped parsley, salt, and pepper. Form into meatballs and brown in a

skillet with olive oil. Add marinara sauce and simmer for 15-20 minutes until meatballs are cooked through.

Vegetable and Tofu Stir-Fry

Ingredients:
Firm tofu, broccoli, bell peppers, snap peas, carrots, garlic, ginger, soy sauce, sesame oil, cornstarch, salt, pepper.

To Prepare :
Press tofu to remove excess water, then cut into cubes. In a pan, stir-fry tofu with chopped vegctables, minced garlic, and grated ginger. In a small bowl, mix soy sauce, sesame oil, and cornstarch to make a sauce. Add the sauce to the stir-fry and cook until vegetables are tender.

Baked Cod with Mediterranean Salsa

Ingredients:
Cod fillets, cherry tomatoes, cucumber, red onion, Kalamata olives, parsley, lemon juice, olive oil, salt, pepper.

To Prepare :

Preheat the oven to 400°F (200°C). Rub cod fillets with olive oil, salt, and pepper. Bake for 12-15 minutes until cooked through. Meanwhile, prepare the salsa by combining diced cherry tomatoes, cucumber, red onion, chopped Kalamata olives, chopped parsley, lemon juice, and olive oil. Serve cod topped with Mediterranean salsa.

Stuffed Bell Peppers with Ground Beef and Rice

Ingredients:

Bell peppers, ground beef, rice, onion, garlic, diced tomatoes, tomato sauce, Worcestershire sauce, Italian seasoning, salt, pepper.

To Prepare :

Preheat the oven to 375°F (190°C). Cook rice according to package instructions. In a skillet, brown ground beef with diced onion and minced garlic. Stir in cooked rice, diced tomatoes, tomato sauce, Worcestershire sauce, Italian seasoning, salt, and pepper. Cut off the bell peppers' tops and extract the seeds. Stuff peppers with beef and rice mixture. Bake peppers for 25 to 30 minutes, or until soft.

Lemon Garlic Shrimp with Zucchini Noodles

Ingredients:
Shrimp, zucchini, garlic, lemon, olive oil, parsley, salt, pepper.

To Prepare :
Using a spiralizer, create zucchini noodles (zoodles). Minced garlic should be sautéed in olive oil in a skillet until aromatic. Add shrimp and cook until pink and opaque. Toss in zucchini noodles, lemon juice, chopped parsley, salt, and pepper. Cook until zucchini noodles are tender.

Greek Yogurt Chicken Salad

Ingredients:
Cooked chicken breast, Greek yogurt, celery, grapes, almonds, lemon juice, dill, salt, pepper.

To Prepare :

Shred cooked chicken breast and place in a bowl. Add Greek yogurt, diced celery, halved grapes, chopped almonds, lemon juice, chopped dill, salt, and pepper. Mix until well combined. Serve on a bed of lettuce or whole grain bread.

Vegetable Frittata

Ingredients:

Eggs, bell peppers, spinach, onion, cherry tomatoes, feta cheese, olive oil, salt, pepper.

To Prepare :

Preheat the oven to 350°F (175°C). In a skillet, sauté diced bell peppers and onion until softened. Add spinach and cook until wilted. In a bowl, whisk eggs with salt and pepper. Pour egg mixture into the skillet and top with halved cherry tomatoes and crumbled feta cheese. Bake for 20-25 minutes until set.

Stuffed Acorn Squash with Quinoa and Cranberries

Ingredients:

Acorn squash, quinoa, dried cranberries, pecans, onion, garlic, vegetable broth, maple syrup, cinnamon, nutmeg, salt, pepper.

To Prepare :

Preheat the oven to 375°F (190°C). Cut the acorn squash in half, then take out the seeds. Roast in the oven for 30 minutes. Meanwhile, cook quinoa according to package instructions. Diced onion and minced garlic should be cooked till tender in a skillet. Stir in cooked quinoa, dried cranberries, chopped pecans, vegetable broth, maple syrup, cinnamon, nutmeg, salt, and pepper. Stuff the roasted acorn squash halves with the quinoa mixture. Bake for an additional 20 minutes.

Mushroom and Spinach Stuffed Chicken Breast

Ingredients:

Chicken breast, mushrooms, spinach, garlic, mozzarella cheese, olive oil, salt, pepper.

To Prepare :

Preheat the oven to 375°F (190°C). In a skillet, sauté sliced mushrooms with minced garlic until softened. Add chopped spinach and cook until wilted. Butterfly chicken breast and stuff with sautéed mushrooms, spinach, and shredded mozzarella cheese. Secure with toothpicks if needed. Season with salt and pepper. Bake for 25-30 minutes until chicken is cooked through.

Black Bean and Corn Salad

Ingredients:

Black beans, corn, red bell pepper, cherry tomatoes, red onion, cilantro, lime juice, olive oil, cumin, chili powder, salt, pepper.

To Prepare :

Rinse and drain black beans and corn. In a bowl, combine black beans, corn, diced red bell pepper, halved cherry tomatoes, diced red onion, chopped cilantro, lime juice, olive oil, cumin, chili powder, salt, and pepper. Toss until well combined.

Sweet Potato and Turkey Chili

Ingredients:
Ground turkey, sweet potatoes, onion, garlic, diced tomatoes, tomato sauce, black beans, chili powder, cumin, paprika, salt, pepper.

To Prepare :
In a large pot, brown ground turkey with diced onion and minced garlic. Add diced sweet potatoes, diced tomatoes, tomato sauce, drained black beans, chili powder, cumin, paprika, salt, and pepper. Simmer for 20-25 minutes until sweet potatoes are tender and flavors are combined.

Zucchini Lasagna

Ingredients:
Zucchini, ground beef, marinara sauce, ricotta cheese, mozzarella cheese, Parmesan cheese, garlic powder, Italian seasoning, salt, pepper.

To Prepare :
Preheat the oven to 375°F (190°C). Slice zucchini lengthwise into thin strips. In a skillet, brown ground beef and season with garlic powder, Italian seasoning, salt, and pepper. Line

a baking dish's bottom with marinara sauce. Layer zucchini strips, ground beef mixture, ricotta cheese, and shredded mozzarella cheese. Repeat layers until ingredients are used up. Top with grated Parmesan cheese. Bake for half an hour while covered with foil. Remove foil and bake for an additional 10-15 minutes until bubbly and golden.

Chicken and Vegetable Skewers

Ingredients:
Chicken breast, bell peppers, zucchini, cherry tomatoes, red onion, olive oil, garlic powder, paprika, salt, pepper.

To Prepare :
Cut chicken breast into cubes. Thread chicken cubes onto skewers alternating with chunks of bell peppers, zucchini slices, cherry tomatoes, and red onion wedges. Brush skewers with olive oil and sprinkle with garlic powder, paprika, salt, and pepper. Grill skewers over medium heat for 8-10 minutes per side until chicken is cooked through and vegetables are tender.

Cauliflower Rice Stir-Fry with Shrimp

Ingredients:
Cauliflower, shrimp, bell peppers, broccoli, carrots, peas, soy sauce, garlic, ginger, sesame oil, salt, pepper.

To Prepare :
Pulse cauliflower florets in a food processor until they resemble rice grains. In a pan, stir-fry shrimp with chopped bell peppers, broccoli florets, sliced carrots, and peas. Add minced garlic and grated ginger. Stir in cauliflower rice and cook until tender. Add salt, pepper, sesame oil, and soy sauce for seasoning.

Vegetarian Lentil Sloppy Joes

Ingredients:
Lentils, onion, bell peppers, tomato sauce, Worcestershire sauce, apple cider vinegar, mustard, brown sugar, chili powder, garlic powder, salt, pepper.

To Prepare :
Prepare lentils as directed on the box. In a skillet, sauté diced onion and bell peppers until

softened. Stir in cooked lentils, tomato sauce, Worcestershire sauce, apple cider vinegar, mustard, brown sugar, chili powder, garlic powder, salt, and pepper. Simmer for 10-15 minutes until flavors are combined and sauce thickens. Serve on whole wheat buns.

Broccoli and Cheddar Quiche

Ingredients:
Pie crust, broccoli, cheddar cheese, eggs, milk, onion, garlic, salt, pepper.

To Prepare :
Preheat the oven to 375°F (190°C). Press pie crust into a pie dish. Blanch broccoli florets in boiling water for 2 minutes, then drain and chop. In a bowl, whisk together eggs, milk, minced garlic, salt, and pepper. Stir in chopped broccoli, grated cheddar cheese, and diced onion. Pour mixture into the pie crust. Bake for 30-35 minutes until the quiche is set and golden brown.

Cabbage and Sausage Skillet

Ingredients:
Cabbage, turkey sausage, onion, garlic, apple cider vinegar, Dijon mustard, paprika, salt, pepper.

To Prepare :
Slice cabbage and turkey sausage. In a skillet, brown turkey sausage with diced onion and minced garlic. Add sliced cabbage and cook until softened. Stir in apple cider vinegar, Dijon mustard, paprika, salt, and pepper. Cook for an additional 5 minutes until flavors are combined.

Honey Garlic Glazed Salmon

Ingredients:
Salmon fillets, honey, soy sauce, garlic, ginger, olive oil, salt, pepper.

To Prepare :
Preheat the oven to 400°F (200°C). Combine the soy sauce, honey, olive oil, grated ginger, chopped garlic, and salt & pepper in a small bowl. Place salmon fillets on a baking sheet lined with parchment paper. Brush salmon with

honey garlic glaze. Bake for 12-15 minutes until salmon is cooked through.

Eggplant Parmesan

Ingredients:
Eggplant, marinara sauce, mozzarella cheese, Parmesan cheese, breadcrumbs, eggs, garlic powder, Italian seasoning, salt, pepper.

To Prepare :
Preheat the oven to 375°F (190°C). Slice eggplant into rounds. Dip eggplant slices in beaten eggs, then coat in a mixture of breadcrumbs, garlic powder, Italian seasoning, salt, and pepper. Arrange breaded eggplant slices on a baking sheet lined with parchment paper. Bake for 20-25 minutes until golden brown. In a baking dish, layer marinara sauce, baked eggplant slices, mozzarella cheese, and Parmesan cheese. Repeat layers. Bake for an additional 15-20 minutes until bubbly and golden.

Shrimp and Avocado Salad

Ingredients:

Shrimp, avocado, mixed greens, cherry tomatoes, cucumber, red onion, lemon juice, olive oil, salt, pepper.

To Prepare :

Cook shrimp until pink and opaque. In a large bowl, toss mixed greens with halved cherry tomatoes, diced cucumber, sliced red onion, cooked shrimp, diced avocado, lemon juice, olive oil, salt, and pepper.

Taco-Stuffed Peppers

Ingredients:

Bell peppers, ground turkey, black beans, corn, diced tomatoes, chili powder, cumin, garlic powder, onion powder, salt, pepper, shredded cheese, cilantro (optional).

To Prepare :

Preheat the oven to 375°F (190°C). Cut off the bell peppers' tops and extract the seeds. In a skillet, brown ground turkey and drain excess fat. Stir in black beans, corn, diced tomatoes, chili powder, cumin, garlic powder, onion powder, salt, and pepper. Fill each bell pepper with turkey mixture and top with shredded cheese. Bake peppers for 25 to 30 minutes, or until soft. Garnish with chopped cilantro if desired.

Mango Salsa Chicken

Ingredients:
Chicken breasts, mango, red bell pepper, red onion, cilantro, lime juice, olive oil, salt, pepper.

To Prepare:
Sprinkle chicken breasts with salt and pepper. Grill or pan-sear chicken until cooked through. In a bowl, combine diced mango, diced red bell pepper, diced red onion, chopped cilantro, lime juice, and olive oil to make the salsa. Serve grilled chicken topped with mango salsa.

Lemon Herb Baked Cod

Ingredients:
Cod fillets, lemon, garlic, fresh herbs (such as parsley, dill, or thyme), olive oil, salt, pepper.

To Prepare :

Preheat the oven to 375°F (190°C). Place cod fillets on a baking sheet lined with parchment paper. Drizzle with olive oil and lemon juice. Sprinkle minced garlic and chopped fresh herbs over the top. Season with salt and pepper. Bake for 15-20 minutes until the fish is cooked through and flakes easily with a fork.

Roasted Brussels Sprouts with Bacon

Ingredients:

Brussels sprouts, bacon, olive oil, garlic powder, salt, pepper.

To Prepare :

Preheat the oven to 400°F (200°C). Trim ends of Brussels sprouts and cut in half. Mix garlic powder, salt, pepper, and olive oil with Brussels sprouts. In an equal layer, spread out onto a baking sheet. Top with chopped bacon. Roast for 25-30 minutes, stirring halfway through, until Brussels sprouts are tender and caramelized.

Turkey and Vegetable Stir-Fry

Ingredients:
Ground turkey, bell peppers, broccoli, carrots, snap peas, onion, garlic, ginger, soy sauce, sesame oil, rice vinegar, honey, cornstarch, olive oil, salt, pepper.

To Prepare:
In a bowl, whisk together soy sauce, sesame oil, rice vinegar, honey, and cornstarch to make the sauce. Heat the olive oil in a big skillet or wok over medium-high heat. Add ground turkey and cook until browned. Add diced bell peppers, broccoli florets, sliced carrots, snap peas, diced onion, minced garlic, and grated ginger. Stir-fry until vegetables are tender-crisp. Pour sauce over the turkey and vegetables. Cook, stirring constantly, until sauce thickens. Serve over cooked rice or quinoa.

Mediterranean Quinoa Salad

Ingredients:
Quinoa, cucumber, cherry tomatoes, Kalamata olives, red onion, feta cheese, fresh parsley, lemon juice, olive oil, salt, pepper.

To Prepare :

Cook quinoa according to package instructions and let cool. In a large bowl, combine cooked quinoa, diced cucumber, halved cherry tomatoes, chopped Kalamata olives, diced red onion, crumbled feta cheese, and chopped fresh parsley. Drizzle with lemon juice and olive oil. Season with salt and pepper. Toss to combine.

Turkey and Vegetable Soup

Ingredients:

Ground turkey, onion, celery, carrots, garlic, diced tomatoes, low-sodium chicken broth, Italian seasoning, bay leaf, salt, pepper, olive oil.

To Prepare :

Heat the olive oil in a big pot over medium heat. Add diced onion, celery, and carrots. Cook until softened. Add minced garlic and cook until fragrant. Add ground turkey and cook until browned. Stir in diced tomatoes, chicken broth, Italian seasoning, bay leaf, salt, and pepper. After bringing to a boil, lower the heat, and simmer for 20 to 25 minutes. Remove bay leaf before serving.

Stuffed Portobello Mushrooms with Quinoa and Spinach

Ingredients:

Portobello mushrooms, quinoa, spinach, onion, garlic, Parmesan cheese, olive oil, balsamic vinegar, salt, pepper.

To Prepare :

Preheat the oven to 375°F (190°C). Remove stems from portobello mushrooms and scrape out the gills. Place mushrooms on a baking sheet. Cook quinoa according to package instructions. Diced onion and minced garlic should be cooked in a skillet till they are tender. Add chopped spinach and cook until wilted. Stir in cooked quinoa and grated Parmesan cheese. Spoon quinoa mixture into the mushroom caps. Drizzle with olive oil and balsamic vinegar. Bake for 20-25 minutes until mushrooms are tender.

Honey Mustard Baked Chicken

Ingredients:

Chicken breasts, Dijon mustard, honey, garlic, olive oil, salt, pepper, fresh herbs (such as thyme or rosemary).

To Prepare :

Preheat the oven to 375°F (190°C). In a bowl, whisk together Dijon mustard, honey, minced garlic, olive oil, salt, and pepper to make the marinade. Place chicken breasts in a baking dish. Pour marinade over the chicken, turning to coat evenly. Bake the chicken for 25 to 30 minutes, or until the juices run clear and the chicken is cooked through. Garnish with fresh herbs before serving.

Spinach and Mushroom Quesadillas

Ingredients:

Flour tortillas, spinach, mushrooms, onion, garlic, shredded cheese (such as mozzarella or cheddar), olive oil, salt, pepper.

To Prepare :

In a skillet, sauté sliced mushrooms with diced onion and minced garlic until softened. Add spinach and cook until wilted. Season with salt and pepper. Lay a flour tortilla flat and sprinkle shredded cheese on one half. Top with the spinach and mushroom mixture. To conceal the filling, fold the tortilla in half. Repeat with remaining tortillas. In a skillet over medium heat, warm the olive oil. Cook quesadillas for 2-3 minutes per side until golden and cheese is melted.

Greek Chicken Pita Wraps

Ingredients:

Chicken breast, Greek seasoning blend, pita bread, tzatziki sauce, cucumber, tomato, red onion, feta cheese, fresh parsley, olive oil, salt, pepper.

To Prepare :

Season chicken breast with Greek seasoning blend. Grill or pan-sear chicken until cooked through. Slice chicken into strips. Use a grill or oven to reheat pita bread. Spread tzatziki sauce on each pita. Top with sliced chicken, diced cucumber, diced tomato, thinly sliced red onion, crumbled feta cheese, and chopped fresh parsley. Sprinkle it with salt and pepper and drizzle with olive oil. Wrap and serve.

Sesame Ginger Tofu Stir-Fry

Ingredients:

Firm tofu, bell peppers, broccoli, snap peas, carrots, onion, garlic, ginger, soy sauce, sesame oil, rice vinegar, honey, cornstarch, sesame seeds, olive oil, salt, pepper.

To Prepare :

Press tofu to remove excess water, then cut into cubes. In a bowl, whisk together soy sauce, sesame oil, rice vinegar, honey, and cornstarch to make the sauce. In a large skillet or wok, heat the olive oil over medium-high heat. Add tofu cubes and cook until golden brown on all sides. Remove tofu from the skillet. In the same skillet, add more olive oil if needed and stir-fry sliced bell peppers, broccoli florets, snap peas, thinly sliced carrots, and diced onion until tender-crisp. Return tofu to skillet and pour sauce over tofu and vegetables. Cook, stirring constantly, until sauce thickens. Garnish with sesame seeds before serving.

Caprese Stuffed Chicken

Ingredients:
Chicken breasts, mozzarella cheese, tomato, fresh basil leaves, balsamic glaze, olive oil, salt, pepper.

To Prepare :
Preheat the oven to 375°F (190°C). Cut a slit horizontally in each chicken breast to create a pocket. Stuff each pocket with sliced mozzarella cheese, sliced tomato, and fresh basil leaves. Drizzle with balsamic glaze and olive oil. Season with salt and pepper. Bake for 25 to 30 minutes, or until the cheese is bubbling and melted and the chicken is thoroughly cooked.

Quinoa-Stuffed Bell Peppers

Ingredients:
Bell peppers, quinoa, black beans, corn, diced tomatoes, chili powder, cumin, garlic powder, onion powder, salt, pepper, shredded cheese, cilantro (optional).

To Prepare :

Preheat the oven to 375°F (190°C). Trim the bell peppers' tops and take out the seeds. Cook quinoa according to package instructions. In a bowl, combine cooked quinoa, rinsed black beans, corn, diced tomatoes, chili powder, cumin, garlic powder, onion powder, salt, and pepper. Fill each bell pepper with quinoa mixture. Top with shredded cheese. Bake peppers for 25 to 30 minutes, or until soft. Garnish with chopped cilantro if desired.

Tuna and White Bean Salad

Ingredients:

Canned tuna, white beans, cherry tomatoes, cucumber, red onion, Kalamata olives, fresh parsley, lemon juice, olive oil, salt, pepper.

To Prepare :

Drain canned tuna and white beans. In a large bowl, combine flaked tuna, white beans, halved cherry tomatoes, diced cucumber, thinly sliced red onion, sliced Kalamata olives, and chopped fresh parsley. Drizzle with lemon juice and olive oil. Season with salt and pepper. Toss to combine.

Turkey Meatballs with Marinara Sauce

Ingredients:
Ground turkey, breadcrumbs, egg, garlic, onion, Parmesan cheese, Italian seasoning, salt, pepper, olive oil, marinara sauce.

To Prepare :
Preheat the oven to 375°F (190°C). In a bowl, combine ground turkey, breadcrumbs, beaten egg, minced garlic, diced onion, grated Parmesan cheese, Italian seasoning, salt, and pepper. Mix until well combined. Form mixture into meatballs and arrange on a parchment paper-lined baking sheet. Bake for 20-25 minutes until cooked through. Serve with marinara sauce.

Stuffed Acorn Squash with Quinoa and Cranberries

Ingredients:

Acorn squash, quinoa, dried cranberries, pecans, onion, garlic, sage, olive oil, salt, pepper.

To Prepare :

Preheat the oven to 400°F (200°C). Cut acorn squash in half lengthwise and scoop out seeds. Brush cut sides with olive oil and season with salt and pepper. Place squash halves cut-side down on a baking sheet lined with parchment paper. Roast for 25-30 minutes until tender. Cook quinoa according to package instructions. Simmer chopped onion and minced garlic in a skillet until they are tender. Stir in cooked quinoa, dried cranberries, chopped pecans, and chopped fresh sage. Season with salt and pepper. Fill each roasted squash half with quinoa mixture.

Zucchini Noodles with Pesto and Cherry Tomatoes

Ingredients:
Zucchini, cherry tomatoes, pesto sauce, olive oil, salt, pepper, Parmesan cheese.

To Prepare :
Using a spiralizer, spiralize zucchini into noodles. In a skillet over medium heat, warm the olive oil. Add spiralized zucchini noodles and halved cherry tomatoes. Cook for 3-5 minutes until zucchini noodles are tender. Stir in pesto sauce until evenly coated. Season with salt and pepper. Serve topped with grated Parmesan cheese.

Salmon and Asparagus Foil Packets

Ingredients:
Salmon fillets, asparagus spears, lemon, garlic, fresh dill, olive oil, salt, pepper.

To Prepare :
Preheat the oven to 375°F (190°C). Cut four sheets of aluminum foil. Place a salmon fillet in

the center of each foil sheet. Season salmon with salt, pepper, minced garlic, and chopped fresh dill. Arrange asparagus spears around the salmon. Drizzle with olive oil and squeeze lemon juice over the top. Fold the edges of the foil over the salmon and asparagus to create a packet. Bake for 15-20 minutes until salmon is cooked through and asparagus is tender.

Vegetarian Chili

Ingredients:
Kidney beans, black beans, diced tomatoes, corn, onion, bell peppers, garlic, chili powder, cumin, paprika, olive oil, salt, pepper.

To Prepare :
Heat the olive oil in a big pot over medium heat. Add the minced garlic, diced onion, and diced bell peppers. Cook until softened. Stir in kidney beans, black beans, diced tomatoes, corn, chili powder, cumin, paprika, salt, and pepper. Simmer for 20 to 25 minutes, stirring from time to time. Serve hot.

Baked Stuffed Chicken Breast with Spinach and Feta

Ingredients:
Olive oil, salt, pepper, garlic, feta cheese, spinach, and chicken breasts.

To Prepare :
Preheat the oven to 375°F (190°C). Pound chicken breasts to an even thickness. Heat the olive oil in a pan over medium heat. Add minced garlic and cook until fragrant. Add chopped spinach and cook until wilted. Take off the heat and mix in the feta cheese crumbles. Spread spinach and feta mixture evenly over each chicken breast. Roll up chicken breasts and secure with toothpicks. Place in a baking dish. Add a drizzle of olive oil and season with pepper and salt. Bake for 25-30 minutes until chicken is cooked through.

Lentil and Vegetable Soup

Ingredients:
Green lentils, carrots, celery, onion, garlic, diced tomatoes, vegetable broth, bay leaf, thyme, olive oil, salt, pepper.

To Prepare :

Rinse lentils and set aside. Olive oil should be heated over medium heat in a big pot. Add the diced carrots, celery, and onion. Cook until softened. Add minced garlic and cook until fragrant. Stir in lentils, diced tomatoes, vegetable broth, bay leaf, and thyme. When lentils are tender, reduce heat and simmer for 30 to 35 minutes after bringing to a boil. Season with salt and pepper. Remove bay leaf before serving.

Chicken and Vegetable Sheet Pan Dinner

Ingredients:
Chicken thighs, baby potatoes, carrots, broccoli florets, red bell pepper, onion, garlic, olive oil, Italian seasoning, salt, pepper.

To Prepare :
Preheat the oven to 400°F (200°C). Place chicken thighs, baby potatoes, sliced carrots, broccoli florets, diced red bell pepper, and sliced onion on a large sheet pan. Add a drizzle of olive oil and season with salt, pepper, and Italian seasoning. Toss to coat evenly. Arrange

ingredients in a single layer on the sheet pan. Bake for 25 to 30 minutes, or until the veggies are soft and the chicken is cooked through.

Pasta Primavera

Ingredients:
Pasta (such as spaghetti or fettuccine), zucchini, yellow squash, bell peppers, cherry tomatoes, garlic, olive oil, Parmesan cheese, fresh basil, salt, pepper.

To Prepare :
Prepare pasta as directed on the package. Drain and set aside. In a big skillet, warm up the olive oil over medium heat. Add sliced zucchini, sliced yellow squash, sliced bell peppers, halved cherry tomatoes, and minced garlic. Cook until vegetables are tender. Add cooked pasta to the skillet and toss to combine. Season with salt and pepper. Serve topped with grated Parmesan cheese and chopped fresh basil.

Salmon Cakes with Dill Sauce

Ingredients:

Canned salmon, breadcrumbs, egg, onion, garlic, Dijon mustard, fresh dill, lemon juice, olive oil, salt, pepper, Greek yogurt.

To Prepare :

Drain canned salmon and remove any skin and bones. In a bowl, combine salmon, breadcrumbs, beaten egg, diced onion, minced garlic, Dijon mustard, chopped fresh dill, lemon juice, salt, and pepper. Mix until well combined. Shape mixture into patties. In a skillet over medium heat, warm the olive oil. Cook salmon cakes for 3-4 minutes per side until golden brown and cooked through. In a small bowl, mix Greek yogurt with chopped fresh dill and lemon juice to make the sauce. Serve salmon cakes with dill sauce on the side.

MEAL PLAN

Day 1:
- Breakfast: Almonds and sliced strawberries with Greek yogurt.
- Lunch: Grilled chicken salad dressed with a balsamic vinaigrette, cherry tomatoes, cucumbers, and mixed greens.
- Dinner: Baked salmon with steamed broccoli and quinoa

Day 2:
- Breakfast: Oatmeal with sliced banana and walnuts
- Lunch: Turkey and avocado wrap with whole grain tortilla
- Dinner: Brown rice, bell peppers, and snap peas stir-fried tofu.

Day 3:
- Breakfast: Scrambled eggs with spinach and whole grain toast
- Lunch: Mixed green salad on the side and lentil soup.
- Dinner: Baked chicken thighs along with green beans and roasted sweet potatoes.

Day 4:

- Breakfast: Smoothie with spinach, banana, almond milk, and protein powder
- Lunch: Quinoa salad with chickpeas, cherry tomatoes, feta cheese, and lemon vinaigrette
- Dinner: Grilled shrimp skewers with grilled zucchini and couscous

Day 5:

- Breakfast: Cottage cheese with sliced peaches and sunflower seeds
- Lunch: Lettuce wraps with tuna salad and carrot and cucumber sticks.
- Dinner: Turkey meatballs with marinara sauce over spaghetti squash

Day 6:

- Breakfast: Poached eggs and avocado on whole grain bread
- Lunch: Greek salad with feta cheese, grilled chicken, olives, and Greek dressing
- Dinner: Baked cod with roasted asparagus and quinoa pilaf

Day 7:

- Breakfast: Overnight oats topped with mixed berries, chia seeds, and almond milk.
- Lunch: Egg salad sandwich with whole grain bread and carrot sticks
- Dinner: Stir-fried beef with brown rice, broccoli, and bell peppers.

Day 8:

- Breakfast: Yogurt parfait topped with sliced kiwis and granola.
- Lunch: Veggie wrap with hummus, bell peppers, cucumber, and spinach
- Dinner: Grilled steak with roasted Brussels sprouts and mashed cauliflower

Day 9:

- Breakfast: Smoothie bowl with mixed fruit and granola topping
- Lunch: Chicken Caesar salad with romaine lettuce, grilled chicken, Parmesan cheese, and Caesar dressing
- Dinner: Baked tilapia with sautéed spinach and quinoa

Day 10:

- Breakfast: Spinach and mushrooms on top of scrambled tofu.
- Lunch: Caprese salad with sliced tomatoes, fresh mozzarella, basil, and balsamic glaze
- Dinner: Turkey chili with kidney beans, diced tomatoes, and avocado garnish

Day 11:

- Breakfast: Whole grain pancakes with maple syrup and sliced strawberries
- Lunch: Quinoa tabbouleh salad with cucumber, tomatoes, parsley, and lemon dressing
- Dinner: Grilled chicken skewers with grilled zucchini and brown rice

Day 12:

- Breakfast: Black bean, avocado, salsa, and scrambled eggs in a burrito.
- Lunch: Spinach salad with grilled salmon, avocado, almonds, and raspberry vinaigrette
- Dinner: Baked tofu with roasted vegetables and wild rice

Day 13:

- Breakfast: Mango slices and chia seed pudding with coconut milk.
- Lunch: Whole-grain veggie burger topped with tomato, onion, and lettuce
- Dinner: Lemon herb roasted chicken with roasted carrots and quinoa

Day 14:

- Breakfast: Whole grain waffles with Greek yogurt and mixed berries
- Lunch: Turkey and Swiss cheese sandwich on whole grain bread with carrot sticks
- Dinner: Grilled shrimp tacos with cabbage slaw, avocado, and corn tortillas

CONCLUSION

As you reach the end of this cookbook journey, it's important to reflect on the transformational impact of embracing the no gallbladder diet. By incorporating these delicious and nourishing recipes into your daily routine, you've taken proactive steps towards improving your digestive health and overall well-being.

Throughout this cookbook, you've discovered a diverse array of flavorful dishes designed to support your dietary needs without sacrificing taste or satisfaction. From hearty salads to comforting soups, each recipe has been carefully crafted to provide nourishment while minimizing discomfort.

By following the principles of the no gallbladder diet, you've empowered yourself to make informed choices about the foods you consume, allowing you to enjoy meals with confidence and peace of mind.

Whether you're managing symptoms post-surgery or simply seeking to optimize your digestive health, the recipes within these pages offer a roadmap to success.

But beyond the kitchen, this cookbook represents a commitment to self-care and holistic wellness. It's a reminder that prioritizing your health is an ongoing journey—one that requires dedication, mindfulness, and a willingness to explore new possibilities.

As you continue on your culinary adventure, remember to listen to your body and honor its unique needs. Pay attention to how different foods make you feel, and don't be afraid to experiment with new ingredients and flavors.

With each meal, you have the opportunity to nourish not only your body but also your spirit, cultivating a deeper connection to yourself and the world around you.

So, as you embark on this next chapter of your health journey, carry with you the knowledge and wisdom gained from these pages. Embrace the joy of cooking, the pleasure of eating, and the transformative power of nourishing your body from the inside out.

*Here's to your
continued health,
happiness, and vitality.
Bon appétit!*

SHOPPING LIST

1. Lean proteins:
   - Chicken breast
   - Turkey
   - Fish (salmon, cod, tilapia)
   - Tofu
   - Eggs

2. Vegetables:
   - Leafy greens (spinach, kale, lettuce)
   - Broccoli
   - Bell peppers
   - Tomatoes
   - Carrots
   - Cucumbers
   - Zucchini
   - Asparagus
   - Brussels sprouts
   - Mushrooms

3. Fruits:
   - Apples
   - Bananas
   - Berries (strawberries, blueberries, raspberries)
   - Oranges

- Avocado
- Kiwi
- Mango
- Peaches

4. Whole grains:
  - Quinoa
  - Brown rice
  - Oats
  - Whole grain bread
  - Whole grain pasta

5. Legumes:
  - Lentils
  - Chickpeas
  - Black beans
  - Kidney beans

6. Dairy and alternatives:
  - Greek yogurt
  - Almond milk
  - Cottage cheese
  - Feta cheese

7. Nuts and seeds:
  - Almonds
  - Walnuts

- Sunflower seeds
- Chia seeds

8. Healthy fats and oils:
   - Olive oil
   - Avocado oil
   - Coconut oil

9. Herbs and spices:
   - Basil
   - Parsley
   - Garlic
   - Ginger
   - Turmeric
   - Cumin
   - Paprika
   - Black pepper
   - Sea salt

10. Condiments and flavorings:
   - Balsamic vinegar
   - Soy sauce (low-sodium)
   - Lemon juice
   - Mustard
   - Honey
   - Salsa